Managing Alzheimer's and Dementia Behaviors

COMMON SENSE CAREGIVING

GARY JOSEPH LEBLANC

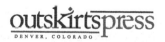

DENVER, COLORADO

Books also by Gary Joseph LeBlanc

Staying Afloat in a Sea of Forgetfulness

While I Still Can
(Co-authored)

Acknowledgments

I would like to give endless thanks to all the readers of my column "Common Sense Caregiving" for the faithful years of endless support and encouragement.

Also, to Brooksville Regional Hospital in Hernando County, Florida for helping and believing in the Alzheimer's/Dementia Hospitalization Wristband Project.

And especially, Holly Beth Michaels who has worked with me on the past three books and has always truly believed in the cause of helping caregivers everywhere.

Table of Contents

CHAPTER 1
Introduction

Ibegan writing this manuscript for the educational program of the Alzheimer's/ Dementia Hospitalization Wristband Project that I initiated. After working on this venture for many years now, I find it has grown near and dear to my heart, becoming somewhat of a passion of mine.

This work was initially designed to be a handbook for all hospital employees to read and discuss, in order to learn better ways of handling patients that suffer from Alzheimer's and other dementia related diseases. However, I soon discovered that every time I would let someone read the unpublished booklet, I heard these familiar words, "You need to do something with this; this could help so many people. . ."

So, this is the primary reason I decided to

rework the book, directing it toward health professionals and family caregivers, keeping it in my traditional "Caregiver Friendly" manner.

My hope is that eventually (soon) all adult care facilities, home care agencies and anyone else who is caring for those that are memory-impaired, will receive in their hands this easy-to-read booklet. If so, they will quickly learn how to deal with certain behavioral situations and become familiar with what the families of these patients are enduring.

Building better communications between the heath professionals and the patients' caregivers is my goal. This also includes the communications between hospitals and patients' living facilities. There are so many cases where the staff of these "homes away from home" are the only advocates the patients have left.

When someone is caring for those suffering from dementia, they cannot move them into their lifestyle; instead they, the caregivers, have to learn how to move into the world of the ones whose minds are afflicted.

"Too often we underestimate the power of touch, a smile, a kind word, a listening ear, an honest compliment or the smallest act of caring, all of which have a potential to turn a life around."

~ Leo Buscaglia

CHAPTER 2
Alzheimer's / Dementia Hospitalization Wristband

My goal is to assure that all patients with Alzheimer's or other dementia related diseases, will experience as calm and unperplexed a stay as is possible during any time spent in a hospital. With this thought in mind we have recently designed a specific wristband which will be fitted to all patients with dementia at the time of their hospital admittance. The band is white with purple lettering, stating: "Alert Advocate."

The very sight of this band will communicate to all hospital staff that these patients are memory-impaired and to approach them with this in mind.

My own personal experience has taught me that it is impossible to identify a memory-impaired person just by sight. I was the primary caregiver for my dad for a decade. He eventually passed away from Alzheimer's, but during the living years, when he was ill, every hospital visit he (we) endured was a complete nightmare. I attempted to remain at his side at all times, knowing I had to be there to be his advocate, but this goal is a difficult one to achieve.

I once took a ten minute break to get some fresh air only to return to find a nurse towering over him, clipboard in hand, impatiently drilling him about his medical prescription history. This poor man couldn't even have told her if he had even taken any pills five minutes ago.

If he had been wearing that particular wristband, it would have alerted her of his memory-impairment, and that he should not be answering important medical questions that could lead to severe complications. Instead, family members or the patients' advocate should be contacted for all medical and personal history.

Oftentimes, serious mis-communications occur between hospital staff and patients' family members who are simply trying to protect their loved ones. It is my hope that hurt feelings and misunderstandings can be avoided when, right from the start, the patients' mental status is made known to staff through the sight of this alerting wristband.

Quite often patients are transported into different departments of the hospital, possibly for x-rays or tests of some kind. The nursing staff that is working on the floor where the patients were first admitted may be aware of their condition, but once they leave that wing the wrist band will do its job, vigilantly alerting every hospital employee of these persons' mental condition.

For many years now I have had the privilege of writing a weekly column on "caregiving for the memory-impaired" in both the Tampa Tribune and the Hernando Today. The notoriety this column affords me means that I hear from caregivers, globally, on a daily basis. They often need to use me as a sounding board, relating horror stories about what their loved ones have endured during their hospital stays.

It's bad enough that these people have been removed from their daily routine; suffering from dementia, they are already drenched in confusion and these hospital stays only serve to exacerbate the situation.

I firmly believe that these wristbands will make their hospital admissions safer and less tormenting for them, their families and for the medical staff.

"Tomorrow is the most important thing in our life. Comes into us at midnight very clean, It's perfect when it arrives and it puts itself in our hands. It hopes we've learned something from yesterday."

~ John Wayne

CHAPTER 3

Warning Signs (Early Symptoms of Dementia)

I f you're thinking it's Friday when it's only Monday, don't panic. This is not a reason to suspect that you're exhibiting signs of Alzheimer's. Most everyone drifts through spells of forgetfulness.

However, if you're worried about yourself, patients or your loved ones, there are several warning signs to watch out for. In the initial stages you might notice there to be a strain when attempting to recall:

- Important dates
- Appointments
- Familiar names

I also recommend watching for certain characteristics, such as:

- Repeatedly asking the same question
- Having a shorter attention-span
- Losing sense of time

Some patients problems manifest themselves in working with numbers, such as being unable to balance a checkbook. They may even scribble a check with the date being off by decades. Such lapses might appear to be simple mistakes made by someone who is merely overtired, but when such blunders occur frequently, that may be a warning signal for concern.

Difficulty with reading may also send up a red flag. For example, not making it past the front page of the newspaper or re-reading the first chapter of a book or even being unable to fill out a questionnaire; these are signs which likely point to the possible loss of a normal attention-span.

When your patients' condition worsens, their excuses will flow like a raging river. Alzheimer's patients are notorious for being amazingly clever at fabricating excuses. Perhaps you'll think their just being stubborn, refusing to perform even simple tasks. Remember, it is less embarrassing for them to just say "No" than to appear foolish.

Next come the accusations. When they misplace items, you or somebody else will undoubtedly be blamed. Expect to see rapidly fluctuating mood changes containing frustration expressed over a simple task or errand.

Often, faltering and struggling for words will emerge later, as the disease advances. Patients may no longer join in conversations or even stop speaking in mid-sentence. You can almost see their gears turning, searching to find a common word. My father often called things by the wrong name like, "Please turn up the radio," when in reality he meant the television.

These are changes you need to begin writing down so you can communicate them to the Head Nurse or attending physician. If a diagnosis is to be Alzheimer's Disease, the sooner it is known the better. Encourage family members to join the staff in creating a care plan tailored specifically for the patient in question.

Please be aware that many of these symptoms could be caused by medications, stress or even depression. This is the reason that it is vitally important at the onset to have the patient given a thorough medical examination. Hopefully the diagnosis won't be anything significant and they will be able to enjoy the "golden years" the way they were meant to be spent.

Many times, however, it takes the initial hospital stay to finally lead them into being correctly diagnosed. So, if you're suspicious that a patient is suffering from signs of dementia, please alert the proper authority.

"It is one of the most beautiful compensations of life that no man can sincerely try to help another without helping himself."

~ Ralph Waldo Emerson

CHAPTER 4
Hospitalization

Let's look again at the havoc that often results from memory-impaired persons spending time in a hospital setting. First of all they have been taken out of their routine. Confusion will multiply about a thousand fold and you (and they) will find yourselves wondering what the heck just happened to them.

My father went through one hospital stay where we couldn't convince him he was even in a hospital. New faces, strange surroundings, beeping equipment only served to overwhelm him the entire time he was there. He was placed in a bed that was on the door side of the room while his roommate concalesced in the bed by the window. A curtain dividing the two beds gave my father almost a "tunnel vision" effect which made matters even worse. When people came to visit the other fellow, all my dad heard were unfamiliar voices which almost drove him mad. He constantly insisted that someone needed to close doors on the other side of the room. (And when I say constantly I mean that literally.) But the problem was, the "doors" didn't even exist.

By the end of the second day his roommate was, understandably, begging to be moved to another room. I privately asked him on his way out what had taken him so long. He answered, "I was trying to be polite, but I just can't take it anymore. I don't know how you do it."

After this gentleman vacated, this left the bed by the window unoccupied. I asked the nurses if it was possible for my father to be moved to the other side of the room. I tried to explain that I believed my father would handle the situation so much better if he could see more of his surroundings. They stared at me as if I was insane. After all, the bed had just been freshly made! Go figure.

At the time loved ones are admitted, caregivers must insist that the hospital staff make a note in big bold letters in their medical chart that these patients are suffering from DEMENTIA and have the "Alert Advocate" wristband placed on them.

Early the next morning I told Dad's doctor that the nurses had refused to move him and explained my theory of why I felt it was important. To my surprise he said, "I'll be right back." Within the hour my dad had a new view, now being able to look out of the window, the door and even into the hallway. It was like the difference between night and day. Although my father was still in mass confusion, now, by being able to see into the corridor, he now had some sense that he actually was in a hospital. His mind was much more at ease as now he was seeing patients pass by in wheelchairs or walking by clutching the backs of their hospital gowns.

During one hospital stay, my father constantly ripped his I.V. out of his arm. It got to the point where already busy nurses from Intensive Care were being brought in to try to locate another vein. I suggested to his nurses that they write on his arm "Do Not Remove," because every time I had asked my father why he kept pulling out his tubing, his response was "No one gave me any instructions." The nursing staff actually laughed at me. But, two days later I came back up from the cafeteria, and sure enough, my father had a pink post it note taped to his arm which said, you guessed it, "Do not remove." My father never pulled his I.V. out again.

Like most other primary caregivers, I knew my "patient" better than anyone, maybe even better than he knew himself.

There are often too many new faces, too many people who don't know how to handle someone with Alzheimer's Disease and too many medical professionals that just won't listen to the caregivers. This is one of the major complaints I hear from caregivers everywhere.

As you can see no one should simply drop Alzheimer's or dementia patients off at the hospital and believe that they're going to be cared for. Someone needs to be there physically and also be their voice, assisting the staff to get to know them.

Every time my father went into the hospital my sister and I would take shifts staying with him. The staff always had plenty of questions and the chance that they would receive the correct answer from him was very slim. If you should observe a patient who does not have an advocate consider speaking with the physician about having a prescribed sitter stay by his or her side, if needed.

In essence, be forewarned that a trip to the hospital for these people only adds additional stress to them, their caregivers and the staff. When the family finally gets them back home it could be days, if not weeks, before they return to any kind of normalcy. I truly believe that, from the trauma of these hospital stays, some patients lose a whole year of what cognitive function they have left.

"I've learned that people will forget what you said, people will forget what you did, but people will never forget how you made them feel."

~ Maya Angelou

CHAPTER 5
The Difference Between Alzheimer's and Dementia

After spending much time conferring with the general public I have come to the conclusion that most people have a hard time distinguishing between Alzheimer's and dementia.

Recently, I was thrilled to read an article by Dr. Robert Stern, Director of The Boston University Alzheimer's Disease Center. Stern simply explained that, "Dementia is a symptom, and Alzheimer's is the cause of the symptom. A good analogy to the term dementia is 'fever.' Fever refers to an elevated temperature, indicating that the person is sick, but it does not touch on any information on what is causing the sickness." So, basically what he's saying is that dementia is not the disease; it is one of the symptoms of the disease.

There are many causes of dementia and some are reversible. But unfortunately, 70-80 percent of all cases occur from Alzheimer's which is not reversible. In fact, it is a fatal disease climbing the charts as one of the leading causes of death.

The word "dementia" has come to replace many old terms such as senility, having senior moments or experiencing a second childhood. It is also important to know that dementia is not necessarily a normal part of aging. If it does present itself, the person showing signs should be checked out thoroughly. The significance of a correct diagnosis could make all the difference in putting the patient on the right track and possibly curing the problem.

Fighting for the cause against Alzheimer's includes educating the public to be aware of all the disabilities involved with the disease. This also means educating the medical community. Over the past several years I have noticed many doctors becoming at ease with the inclination toward diagnosing the patient with Alzheimer's Disease a little too quickly when, in fact, it may actually be a form of dementia that could be reversible.

So remember this; when dealing with Alzheimer's or dementia, beginning with a proper diagnosis is essential so that the patient can immediately be prescribed the correct treatment or therapy and the medical staff and family can plan ahead from this point and get started on the right foot.

"It is curious that physical courage should be so common in the world, and moral courage so rare."

~ Mark Twain

CHAPTER 6
Early-Onset of Alzheimer's

Although symptoms of Alzheimer's Disease has usually been known to appear in people that are in their late sixties or older, there are now an estimated 1/2 million people under the age of sixty-five who have become afflicted with the disease. This is known as "Early-Onset Alzheimer's Disease." Studies show that there are cases of patients in their thirties, but this is extremely rare.

The genetic path of inheritance is much greater in Early-Onset Alzheimer's. Those that have a parent or grandparent who developed the disease at a younger age have a higher risk for contracting it themselves.

When this disease invades so early in life, a number of problems quickly unfold. These newly stricken patients may still be caring for a parent afflicted with the same illness and, meanwhile, may have their own children still living at home. Family members, neighbors and coworkers might ridicule and berate these persons, calling them straight-out lazy, when the fact of the matter is, Alzheimer's has destroyed their motivation and concentration. Commonly, patients experience heavy bouts of depression and frustration. Often, even marital problems develop from being misunderstood and mis-diagnosed.

According to the experts, 80 percent of these patients will lose their employment and their corresponding income.

Alzheimer's Disease is devastating at any age, but it seems to be so much more unfair when it strikes at a younger age. Please be aware that the incident of Early-Onset Alzheimer's is growing at an alarming rate.

The familiar picture of an elderly man or woman, staring blankly out of a window from a wheelchair, is no longer the face of Alzheimer's.

"It's a hard thing to leave any deeply routine life, even if you hate it."

~ John Steinbeck

CHAPTER 7
Routine, Routine, Routine

'Round the clock caring for an Alzheimer's patient over the past has truly unearthed several absolutes; at the very top of the list is routine; a steady, run-of-the-mill lifestyle. In fact, routine is probably wholesome for everyone involved. It might seem boring at times, but if you deal with short-term memory, it will be your greatest friend.

In my experience, I found that maintaining a life of habit eased most anxiety and frustration. For instance, I always tried to serve Dad's breakfast and dinner at the same time every day; I even used a specific blue bowl for his pills each morning and evening. When I didn't, we had a problem: "These aren't the pills I took yesterday." Further, at every mealtime I arranged his silverware in a consistent pattern. Whether I served soft pasta or cup of soup, there was always a knife placed at the same spot on the table.

The same rules applied to his clothing. There was no reason for him to be required to make too many choices. Keeping it simple and having only four or five outfits from which to choose kept things uncomplicated.

Then there were those dreaded doctor visits. These would leave him confused for days! Even so, every two or three months we visited the same waiting room with the same staff but he would still religiously ask, "Have we ever been here before?" By the time we arrived home, he couldn't be convinced that he ever even went! To make matters worse, the following day would find him completely out of sync. First, he would wake up earlier than usual, then at breakfast, he would swear he already ate! He would then claim that he already swallowed his pills; at times becoming straight-out delusional. This may sound minor, but as his caregiver I found this quite disconcerting. Believe me, these things have a way of multiplying. By day's end, he was a complete mess and so was I.

I recall when, one day, Dad had two separate doctor appointments scheduled. This was a variation on an already distressing theme. On the way home he kept insisting I was going the wrong way, while continuously opening the car door as it was moving! I never made that scheduling mistake again.

The more established your patients' life is, the more pleasant yours will be. You still might have to step back and take a few deep breaths every now and then, just to deal with the frustrations. Repeating yourself fifty times a day, answering the same questions over and over and listening to multiple excuses can tend to wear the fabric of anyone's nerves a bit thin.

Patients with Alzheimer's Disease are notorious for covering up and making excuses. In my case, Dad always had a rationalization for something he forgot, or what he thought was a plausible reason for why he didn't recognize someone. Here's an example: an emergency room doctor was asking him basic questions to assess his lucidity. One of the questions happened to be, "Do you know who the president is?" He looked at me, then around the room, saying absolutely nothing. The doctor left the room and closed the curtain. Dad promptly quipped, "This guy calls himself a doctor and he doesn't even know who the president is." We could hear the doctor laughing on the other side of that thin curtain wall. The point I'm making is that my father couldn't even understand why he was being asked these questions, let alone give a correct answer.

Keep telling yourself, "It's not the patient's fault"—because it's not. Keep these beloved victims' lives as uncomplicated as possible. Love them and be their most forbearing friend, enjoying them for as long as you still can.

"When we are no longer able to change a situation . . . We are challenged to change ourselves."

~ *Viktor Frankl*

CHAPTER 8
Redirection

When my father progressed into the last stage of Alzheimer's, redirecting his thoughts became almost impossible.

Previously, I was able to turn his fixation onto a different subject, but in the final stage his delusions and hallucinations became so pronounced that I could only divert his train of thought for a few seconds at a time, at best.

When caring for Alzheimer's patients, you must learn to use redirection as a tool to your advantage. Become attuned to the signs that confusion is about to begin, as it will likely commence to snowball straight into delusion or worse. Use simply phrased words and you may be able to create a u-turn in thought patterns. These are essential skills that I recommend highly that all caregivers master.

When patients begin speaking of topics which

make absolutely no sense, casually interrupt with a quick statement like, "That color looks great on you. You should wear that color more often."

Steering their minds onto subjects they can actually see, smell or touch will save hours of misery for you, thwarting you from having to listen to convoluted chatter. Try handing them something tangible, like two different colored wash cloths; for example a green one and a blue one or any other two items that are similar. Ask them which of the two they like better. It may be an hour before you get an answer, or maybe never. The point is you now have directed their confused thoughts onto another subject. Sometimes if they can actually hold objects in their hands they will be redirected faster and for a longer period.

If they are still able to chew and swallow you might want to try something referred to as "Gum Therapy." It's worth a try. A single stick of chewing gum might land you a peaceful thirty minutes. This might be substituted with hard candy or ice cream. For me, ice cream was like "manna from Heaven;" it often brought me some peace and quiet in seconds.

Let's take a look at a common foe of Alzheimer's

Disease victims; anxiety. It could be playing a significant role in causing severe disorientation. If the patient has already been on a particular anxiety medication for a long period of time, it might be beneficial to discuss with his or her physician the possibility of increasing the dosage or trying something new. However, redirection should always be attempted first.

Many of my father's mornings began with him believing he was on a train. He would ask, "Could you please tell me when the next stop is going to be? I believe that's where I have to get off." When I tried to reassure him that we were home in our own house, his response was, "Come on! I can feel the train moving." It's best to just go along for the ride. The last thing I needed was to get his feathers all ruffled before his day even started.

So, Dear Caregivers, hold on tight. From here on out, the ride may have fewer stops. If a mental image has worked them into a frenzy, chances are it's going to last the entire day. One of the hardest things I dealt with was convincing my father he was home. He constantly wanted to know why he could not go to his parents' house or some other place that he believed was his abode.

Keep in mind that during the last stage of the disease, you'll probably need the minimum of two people to help with the patients you are caring for. Attempting to do everything yourself could erupt into a physical or mental fiasco; probably both. Create a schedule so that you know when relief is coming.

If our loved ones were able, they would surely advise us to take care of ourselves, so that when the inevitable comes to pass, and they die, we will hopefully be able to begin enjoying our own lives again.

"Believe in yourself! Have faith in your abilities! Without a humble but reasonable confidence in your own powers you cannot be successful or happy."

~ Norman Vincent Peale

CHAPTER 9

Learning to Approach Someone with Alzheimer's

By not knowing the correct and pragmatic way to approach a person who has Alzheimer's disease or dementia has caused many family members and old friends to refrain from visiting the ones they love. This is tragic!

It is heartbreaking to watch as loved ones fades away right in front of our very eyes, but in my opinion, not seeing them at all is much worse for all involved. I've had so many different caregivers tell me that their sons or daughters won't visit a parent because they just can't handle seeing them the way they've become, because they're not the same person they used to be.

I believe that once these neglected loved ones are gone, there will remain a certain ruefulness in the heart of the one left behind that may never go away.

It would obviously be best to avoid such a sad state of affairs, so, here are some great tips on how to meet and greet these folks.

First, learn that when you initially walk into a room where they are, enter at a normal pace. Don't rush up on them.

Before you even say a word, make sure they have made visual contact with you. Never come up on them from behind or directly from their side. Greet them face to face with a smile. Mother Teresa was known for saying, "Let us always meet each other with a smile, for the smile is the beginning of love."

Personal space can be a big issue. Give them plenty of breathing room and always stand a step to the right or left, leaving them an escape path. I'm not saying they're going to bolt, but nobody likes to be closed in.

Introduce yourself by name and state your relationship. "Hi, I'm Holly Beth, your daughter." You may hear a loud and snippy remark like, "You're late!" or you may hear nothing at all. In either case it's okay. Whatever you do, don't start off by asking, "Do you remember me?" In fact you're better off making a statement like, "I remember when we . . . ?" This way it's not in the form of a question, as questions tend to raise their anxiety level right off the bat.

If they're sitting down or much shorter than you, try lowering yourself to an equal level. Nobody takes well to someone towering over them. If they're willing to shake your hand and they want to continue to hold it, by all means let them. However, if they don't want to take your hand, respect that as well.

This takes a lot of practice to master, so if doesn't go as planned on the first try, learn from your mistakes and keep trying. You'll get it. Even most of the medical professionals haven't figured it out. You can go into almost any adult living community and witness a CNA walk right up to a patient in a wheelchair and, before making verbal or eye contact, begin to propel them down the hall. This would frighten anyone.

Most of these tips I've just suggested are concerning those who are in the moderate to latter stages of their disease. If they're in the earlier stages, things should be adjusted so they do not become offended.

Make sure that they are always treated with the respect they truly deserve.

"Acting is not about being someone different. It's finding the similarity in what is apparently different, then finding myself in there."

~ Meryl Streep

CHAPTER 10
Adapting to Character

You will discover, as the disease of Alzheimer's progresses, everyone that the patient knows may receive a new identity. Names might change five times or more in a one hour period.

There is no way to prepare yourself ahead of time for the jarring moment when your loved one looks at you and has no recognition of who you are—it's nothing short of heartbreaking! I always tell family members that they're still inside of them, they just can't be retrieved at that moment. It seems to help them a little bit.

There will be moments when, suddenly, he or she will comprehend who you actually are, but these occasions may start becoming few and far between. When those moments do occur, you may observe through their facial expressions, the profound sorrow he or she may feel.

You must accept that it's not their fault. Pursue

the role they believe you to be and assume your new identity. First, you usually become a close relative; brother, sister, uncle, aunt or family member deep from the past. Later you will assume still another role. Names seem to be randomly drawn out of a hat.

My father most often believed I was his dad. I learned to make this work to my advantage. He definitely listened to me with deeper respect. He would ask, "Dad, do I have to take all these pills?" and then I would softly respond, "Yes son, please take them all and don't make me get your mother involved," which really seemed to get his attention. Playing the role can help both parties. I had become Dad 80 percent of the time, brothers and who knows who 15 percent. Being recognized as his son dwindled to a diminishing final 5 percent.

My father, being the oldest of seventeen children in his family would constantly ask for his brother Alfie, who was the second oldest. Well the reality is, Alfie had passed away shortly after WWII. If I even attempted to tell him this, he would become extremely upset, yelling, "How could you people not even tell me about my brother's funeral? I can't believe I missed it."

I learned just to reflexively tell him, "Alfie just left. He said something about he'd be back in the morning."

Go with the flow. Caregiving is extremely demanding when this happens, but by playing along with the current scenario you will be instrumental in comforting and relieving some of the stress. You must learn to quickly adapt—they did. Once again, you can not move them in to your world, you have to move into theirs.

"There is a sacredness in tears. They are not the mark of weakness, but of power. They speak more eloquently than ten-thousand tongues. They are messengers of overwhelming grief . . . and unspeakable love."

~ Washington Irving

CHAPTER 11
Why Don't You See Them? (Hallucinations and Delusions)

At about nine o'clock one morning my dad began showing signs of being delusional and became extremely upset. "They're breaking into the building next door! All the tools behind the building are being stolen!" Over and over Dad insisted upon this, quite loudly, throughout the entire day. The thing is, the other building wasn't even visible from the house, but he insisted that he saw at least five guys "over there" breaking in. Finally, I walked him "over there," across the field. I repeated this walk with him five times in hopes that it would settle him down. At last, around 5:00 p.m., I just couldn't take it anymore. I called my sister and begged her to drop everything she was doing and come over immediately. Upon her arrival she suggested that I should get away and take a break for awhile. I responded that the only thing I wanted to do at that moment was to get some sleep.

Delusional behavior is only one of the cruel effects of Alzheimer's Disease and was one of the hardest for me to bear. At that point, Dad had been suffering from this pillaging disease for practically a decade, and what I've just described is one of its most heartrending facets.

Hallucinations and delusions are two of the most strenuous side effects for caregivers to contend with. You will really need to call upon all of your endurance in order to avoid losing your patience. Exhibiting signs of frustration will only make matters worse.

Years ago, on a Memorial Day weekend, Dad took a gander out the kitchen window and asked, "What are those twenty-five people doing having dinner in our backyard?"

If it happens that your patient truly believes he or she is witnessing something, do not turn it into a debate. Period! Instead, be affirming with, "I just went out and checked. They must have just left." You might have to take a walk outside and circle the house. (At this point you probably need some fresh air and some good ol' dirt kicking anyway.) Whatever you do, don't get into an argument. It will only twist things further and you both will likely be headed for hours of extended madness.

I confess this was one of the most difficult situations I dealt with as caregiver. There were many times it became necessary to call for back up because I couldn't handle Dad's hallucinations one more minute. Like a "horse rode too hard and put up wet," I needed open pasture. Get the point? Alzheimer's patients can use you up.

At this point during this campaign I had considered myself to be a seasoned caregiver, but now it is easy to admit that the mental madness of these hallucinations and delusions will take even the best of us down.

It's amazing that a fallacy may remain in patients' minds sometimes for days, but then something that just happened two minutes ago will no longer exist.

True or not, what they believe they're seeing, smelling or even tasting is as real to them as the ground we're standing on.

"The suspicious mind believes more than it doubts."

~ Eric Hoffer

CHAPTER 12
The Difference Between Hallucinations and Delusions

If you should have experience the illness of loved ones or if you are caring for patients in a health care setting, it is essential that you become their advocate, even more so if they are afflicted with Alzheimer's Disease or some other form of dementia. Being their voice may mean you will have to explain what you believe is ailing them to the Head Nurse or to their physician. This becomes especially important during the latter stages of the disease. You will likely be required to differentiate between symptoms which can appear very similar to one another.

I have discovered two mental conditions which the general public commonly mistake as being the same thing; hallucinations and delusions.

A delusion is a fictional belief about something, someone or even about oneself. For instance, a common delusion that occurs within Alzheimer's patients is the notion that everyone is stealing from them, taking all of their prized possessions. Suspicion and delusions seem to go hand in hand.

Hallucinations, on the other hand, are false perceptions of objects, people or events. They are not only visible to the person experiencing them, but can be heard, smelled and tasted by the patient. They can become very frightening for them and very difficult for caregivers to handle.

Discuss this matter with their physician. There are medications that may help. If these hallucination are scaring your patients and they are building up high levels of anxiety and redirection will not work, their doctor may want to prescribe something that will.

"Keep you face always toward the sunshine—
and shadows will always fall behind you."

~ *Walt Whitman*

CHAPTER 13

Sundown Syndrome (Sundowning and Evening Confusion)

4:45 p.m.—everyone gets a new name, possibly two. My father, who didn't need a clock for this, he went through this change almost every day toward the end of the moderate stage of his battle with Alzheimer's Disease.

Sundown Syndrome—also known as "sundowning"—is a term describing the onset of heavier confusion and intensified agitation. Usually this begins anywhere from late afternoon to dusk. In reality, it could happen anytime throughout the day.

Experts believe that one of the contributing factors is a shift in the biological clock which is caused from the change of daylight to dark. Keeping patients' environment well lit during these hours will help immensely.

Physical and mental exhaustion is one of the biggest culprits. An Alzheimer's patient's day consists of coping with who's who, "where am I," and living in the past. This would mentally drain anyone.

There are days when I swore my father's sundowners would last morning 'til night. I also recall noticing similar reactions on dispiriting rainy days. Once anxiety builds, it's difficult to turn it around. Keep evenings as calm, routine and simple as possible. Just do the best that you can.

"In everyone's life, at some time, our inner fire goes out. It is then burst into flame by an encounter with another human being. We should all be thankful for those people who rekindle the inner spirit."

~ Albert Schweitzer

CHAPTER 14

Don't Turn Off the Light
(Keeping Things Well Lit)

While my dad's Alzheimer's progressed, he insisted on sleeping with a light on in his room. I'm not talking about a night light, but one bright enough with which to read a pocket-sized dictionary! Having his room glaringly illuminated made it easier for him to calculate his surroundings. After all, Alzheimer's patients are likely to start their day off not realizing whose house they're even in.

I placed old family photos along the wall beside Dad's bed. This was to familiarize and comfort him when he first opened his eyes. Photo albums are a great tool to have lying around the home of an Alzheimer's patient. My dad spent hours flipping through the pages of these old photographs; not always remembering the faces from his past but somehow definitely receiving solace during times of confusion.

Even after waking from a catnap in his recliner it became difficult for him to get his bearings.

Try not to change patients' surroundings. Redecorating their home or changing an art piece on the wall can severely disorient them.

I recall an incident where Dad asked me why someone removed the bed from his room. The only change made was clean sheets and a different colored comforter. Minor changes that would normally seem innocuous could send him into a state of confusion. It even caused hallucinations. So keep things simple and well lit. The memory-impaired need their familiar surroundings to remain unchanged.

"Electric communication will never be a substitute for the face of someone who with their soul encourages another person to be brave and true."

~ Charles Dickens

CHAPTER 15
Body Language &
Communication

Once someone is afflicted with Alzheimer's, they will soon begin to lose their communication skills. Unfortunately, it's inevitable. As a caregiver you will need to adjust your communication and speaking techniques throughout the different stages of the disease, adapting to changes as they occur.

Learn to face the patients directly, talking to them as if they're reading your lips. I'll be the first to admit I was guilty of saying something to my dad as I was walking into another room, only to have to return and speak in a more direct manner, making sure he clearly understood me.

Be patient with them and yourself. This matter can get very frustrating and tiresome. Learn to stay away from subjects that might upset them. I won't make a list of what to avoid as this is unique to each individual. You'll know which ones they are; if you don't, you'll quickly figure them out by the responses you get as the days unfold.

In some of the more orthodox crime detective practices of solving mysteries, trained investigators are taught to always concentrate on asking the five W's: who, what, when, where and why. As a caregiver you will soon discover that you too will have a your daily routine involved in the perpetual task of solving many mysteries. But, on the other hand, these are also five words you will want to refrain from using at certain times.

Common sense should be telling you when to back away from any questions which are incorporated with the five W's.

- Who are you upset with?
- What do you think you're doing?
- When are you going to wash up?
- Where do you think you're going?
- Why are you crying?

Yes, there are many other letters in the alphabet besides W's to worry about. The point being, however, that when you see that they are already having difficulties don't begin making inquiries that you know they probably won't be able to answer, likely causing further turmoil. Just use the five W's as a rule of thumb to hold in abeyance in the back of your mind.

The short-term memory will gradually dissipate from the mind of Alzheimer's patients. Whatever happened just a few minutes ago never occurred in the minds of those stricken with the disease. However, the long-term memory survives until the latter stage of the disease.

Caregivers should make it their goal to maintain patients' verbal abilities extending as far into the disease as feasible, because once they stop speaking everything else begins accelerating downhill from that point.

A fellow caregiver once explained to me that her mother is constantly asking if she can move back to her hometown. Her mom believes that everything would go back to the way things were 40 some years ago and she would be living the same lifestyle of her younger days.

Anyone who is caring for those afflicted with Alzheimer's or dementia has heard or will inescapably hear their patients say, "I want to go home! This is a perfect example of an opportunity and need for redirection. This will always be a caregiver's best tool of defense.

Hearing the statement, "I want to go home" should be taken as a forewarning that wandering may be in the near future. In a nonchalant fashion, pay very close attention to these patients until you feel confident that they have moved on to fresh and more pleasant thoughts.

I'm directing this advice to everyone who is involved in the care of the memory-impaired. This includes home health aids, nursing home employees, family members, etc. This is a situation where patients can easily become lost and possibly seriously hurt.

You must also keep in mind that the words "I want to go home," may mean to them something completely different than what you think. The statement could possibly mean that they simply want things to go back to the way they used to be years ago.

The fact that patients are unable to recognize their own surroundings makes things extremely frightening for them. They will wish they were back in the comfort and safety of what they remember to be their own home.

Once again, casual redirection of an Alzheimer's patient's thoughts is something every caregiver needs to master.

Sadly, people suffering from dementia arrive at a point where they can no longer recall many of the facts about their own life, but they seem quite adept at constructing a new reality.

When they say things you know are wrong, learn not to correct them. This only puts them in a state of confusion. Also, keep your statements short and simple, but please don't demean them by speaking to them as if they are children.

If you're giving them instructions, only direct them to do one thing at a time. If you say to them, "You need to wash your hands and brush your teeth so we can go to the doctor," that will be too much for them to absorb. Mention one step at a time. You might even get there sooner.

Eventually you'll start noticing that they won't stay on the same subject very long. They will stop in the middle of a sentence, and then forget what they were saying. Pay close attention to their "body language." You'll soon learn their facial expressions: pain, depression, confusion and love. They're all in there. Be patient and loving. It is as frustrating for them as it is for you, maybe more so.

"We gain strength, and courage, and confidence by each experience in which we really stop to look fear in the face... we must do that which we think we cannot."

~ Eleanor Roosevelt

CHAPTER 16
Dealing with Combative Behavior

When caring for someone who has Alzheimer's Disease or any other kind of dementia, it is most likely that you will have confrontations with them. Some may even lead into dangerous, combative behavior.

The progression of the disease will eventually reach a point where patients will begin to lose their communication skills. This will only increase their level of frustration, which often leads to problems with their conduct.

I do have some good news, however; this only seems to be a phase, but unfortunately, it could last a couple of years.

In my father's case, he wasn't very combative, but he was extremely verbally abusive. In either case, as difficult as it is, we can't take it personally.

Instead we must investigate what caused them to become upset in the first place. Often our patients' behavior is due to an uncomfortable or stressful environment. It's wise to investigate with the "Five W's" again; when, where, who, what and why the incident occurred.

Try putting yourself in their shoes. Be sure to pay close attention to their body language and envisage how they might be feeling. Imagine what they might be trying to express. Then ask yourself what happened just before the behavior problem started.

The next thing you want to ask yourself is, how did you react to the situation? Did your response help things or make them worse?

As a caregiver, you may or may not be able to control the patients' moods swings, but you do have a chance to calm their environment. Look for potential stressors: loud or unidentifiable noises, dim or shadowy lighting or reflecting surfaces. Mirrors have been known to cause severe problems with dementia patients.

Don't confront the person or attempt to discuss their angry behavior. Whatever you do, do not initiate physical contact. This will often backfire on you making matters worst. A time-out may be the best solution for both of you at this point.

Redirection would be my first tool of choice. Pet therapy is another good call. By placing my father's cat in his lap, many hours of peace came into our home. Just make sure that both of you are safe and don't back yourself into a corner.

Most of the time when they strike out, they're not realizing who you actually are. They may be thinking you're a complete stranger. If things turn nasty, leave the room and let them play out their aggression, as long as they are safe.

As I stated earlier, don't take this outrage personally. It is part of the disease and, truthfully, it's not their fault. It's a hard concept to understand but in most cases it's true.

"Rivers know this: there is no hurry. We shall get there some day."

~ A.A. Milne, Winnie-the-Pooh

CHAPTER 17
Patience is a Virtue

Patience is an essential ingredient for being a successful caregiver. In today's swift paced world, it's difficult to discipline oneself to slow down. Before I became my father's primary caregiver I spent many years working two jobs, averaging 13 hours-a-day, plus another two hours behind the wheel going to and fro. When I arrived in the world of caregiving I felt as if I was constantly driving through a school zone! It was quite the culture shock.

When caring for Alzheimer's patients, let yourself become part of their world, instead of trying to move them into yours.

I can't tell you how many mornings I spent trying to get my father ready for a doctor's appointment, finally asking myself, "Could he possibly be moving any slower?" On one occasion

I decided he was trying to set a new Guinness Book World Record for the slowest shave. I was forever calling the doctor's office to inform them we were "running late as usual."

It takes a patient person to provide care when you're still able to move and process your thoughts quickly, but the persons you're caring for cannot. It is understandably difficult to slow life down. I found myself constantly having to remind myself of how important it was not to rush my father because all it ever accomplished was to increase his confusion ten-fold.

Being an impatient caregiver will only fill the room with anxiety and fear for all of you.

Keep your composure. It is not only important when they're moving in slow motion, but it also has much to do with keeping your cool while they're asking you the same question for the thirtieth time. Learning to bite your tongue and refrain from yelling, "I just told you that" all falls into the same category: forbearance. If you catch yourself speaking in an angry voice take a step outside and breathe in some fresh air and kick a little dirt around. You must remain diligent in your awareness of knowing when you're about to lose your patience. When you feel this beginning to happen more and more often, it's only common sense to recognize this as a sign that you are in dire need of some respite care.

Patience is the state of endurance under extremely trying circumstances, and there's no better example of these circumstances than when caregiving.

I don't know who first said, "Patience is a virtue," but I believe they might have been a caregiver at one point in their life.

"But I have promises to keep, and miles to go before I sleep, and miles to go before I sleep."

~ Robert Frost

CHAPTER 18
A Caregiver's Promise

When caring for Alzheimer's patients, you may hear them utter things that are so far off the wall that there's no making heads nor tails of what they're talking about. But keep in mind, through all this chatter, you might come across some things said that should never be repeated to anyone.

"Patient confidentiality" is a trust and bond that should be taken seriously by everyone who works in the healthcare profession. This rule should even apply to the person doing the much needed job of housekeeping.

Privacy is a public right and we, as a society, have an ethical obligation to protect the memory-impaired. These patients could be having what seems like a normal conversation with just anyone when suddenly they become paranoid that everyone is against them and stealing all their belongings. Next they will demand that you go out to their back yard and start digging up coffee cans full of money they buried behind the big oak tree. Chances are the money was already dug up some twenty years ago, if there ever was any in the first place that is.

There can always be an exception to the rule. In a situation like this, the patients' legal guardian or their power of attorney should be informed. But remember; it may not just have to do with money. I have heard several stories of patients burying their guns in the backyard. Obviously, this information needs to be investigated immediately as well.

Another frequent problem when dealing with Alzheimer's patients is that they rarely give the same answer to a question two times in a row. So, when they claim they're having chest pains or some other types of body aches they should be taken seriously and their physician immediately notified. Don't ignore other complaints but use discretion in discerning the severity.

And still another significant concern is "identity theft." Just in the United States alone, an estimated 13.3 people have their identity stolen every minute. It's part of the caregiver's job to make sure that patients aren't being forgetful or foolishly mishandling their wallet or purse. The responsibility of keeping them safe involves more than just their physical well being.

Even when caregivers are out enjoying what little social life they have, they must remain on their toes and not spill out any personal information that could cause harm to the patients. There's always someone out there waiting to prey on people who are most vulnerable. There's an old saying, "between you and me and the lamppost." Well, leave the lamppost and the extra person out of this.

If unwarranted questions are asked about these patients, simply answer, "It would be inappropriate for me to answer that."

Today's technology lends itself to the thievery of personal information. If faxing important documents, be sure to remove the original papers from the machine. Also, sensitive e-mails should always be deleted.

I personally know how stressful and demanding the job of being a caregiver is and I hate to add more worries on top of the ones you already have. But these people are depending on you and if that bond of trust becomes compromised, patients may start holding back vital information such as some of the severe symptoms they're experiencing.

A true caregiver/patient relationship must be built on honest-to-goodness trust. Stay faithful to them; loyalty is everything.

CPSIA information can be obtained at www.ICGtesting.com
Printed in the USA
BVOW09s0954151214

379123BV00004B/56/P